HIGH CARB

LIVE A HAPPY, ENERGETIC, AND PEACEFUL LIFE NOW: WHY LOW-CARB DIETS ARE NOT A SOLUTION

BY

BASTIEN DARROW

Copyright © 2015

INTRODUCTION

There are a many diets that are out there which describe the evils of eating carbs and how they are causing you to be fat and increase your chances of getting health issues. Unfortunately, this information is backwards and is causing you to become sick. In fact, those who eat too much fat are the ones who are becoming unhealthy and will fight with obesity and other issues.

This guidebook is going to discuss some of the benefits that you can get when you consume healthy carbs in your diet. You will learn the differences in the types of carbs, the benefits of vegan diets, how fat can harm you, and comparison about societies around the world who eat more carbs versus those who eat more fat.

Carbs are not the enemy with your diet; eating the right kinds and amounts of foods are important in keeping healthy. Use this guidebook to get started on the right track to losing weight and staying healthy for the long term.

TABLE OF CONTENTS

Chapter 1. Introduction to Carbs

Carbs have gotten a bad name in today's health industry. Many diets proclaim that eating carbs s going to ruin your health and make you feel miserable. There are diet plans that ask you to pretty much eliminate the carbs you are consuming in order to be healthy. But are carbs really that bad?

This chapter is going to discuss this in detail and explain the differences between good carbs and bad carbs in your diet.

WHY CARBS ARE CONSIDERED BAD

It is often believed that carbs are unhealthy and that you should avoid them as much as possible. This thought process was begun not due to carbs being bad, but the types of carbs and the way that people eat carbs that is bad.

For example, spending all day eating donuts is not the same as having a nice whole wheat pasta with lots f veggies. Both are going to give you a good dose of carbs, but the first option is going to make you feel sick and raise your blood sugar levels while the other will leave you feeling full and satisfied.

Your body needs carbs; the issue comes when you are eating the wrong kinds of carbs. Simple carb are going to make your blood sugar spike real high, but soon it will crash. When this crash occurs, you will be hungry and not feel so good anymore, even though you might have just consumed a large meal. Over time, this spike and then drop in blood sugar levels can lead to health issues, such as diabetes and heart issues. With this information, it is no surprise that some people feel it is completely better to eliminate carbs from their diet to avoid the issues.

But your body needs the carbs in order to stay healthy and happy. Eating the right carbs will provide the body with the energy that it needs to keep going and will not cause the large spikes in sugar that simple carbs do. These are known as complex carbs and should be included in your daily diet.

The differences between the kinds of carbs you should consume will be discussed further in the next section.

THE DIFFERENT KINDS OF CARBS

There are two main types of carbs that you can consume in your food and each of them will react in a different way in your body. These two main types of carbs include simple carbs and complex carbs.

Simple cars are the sugars such as ones found in milk products, milk, vegetables, and fruits. The carbs that are found in these foods are often low in nutrients but high in simple sugars, the ones that are known to rise up your blood sugar levels. It is best to try and avoid these kinds of carbs as much as possible or to choose options that do not contain as much of the simple carbs. For example, choosing an option such as brown sugar, molasses, syrup, and anything with high fructose corn syrup in it is going to provide you with fewer nutrients compared to choosing fruits and vegetables. Both will contain simple carbs, but the fruits and vegetables will provide you with more nutrients in addition to the carbs to help keep your sugar levels in check.

Complex carbs would include starch as well as dietary fiber. Starch is a nutrient that is going to need to go through digestion in order to use it as a source for glucose. This means that you will be taking longer to digest up the starch and it will keep you feeling fuller for longer and can keep the blood sugar levels more in check. They still may rise a bit, but instead of doing it all at once and then crashing, the release of the carbs will be slower so the rise and fall will be steadier.

Some foods that you can eat that contain starch in them would include vegetables such as corn, peas, dry beans, and potatoes, grains, breads, cereals, whole grain foods, and some fruits.

You should also include fiber into your diet. This is a great carb because it is going to keep the hunger pains away even if you only eat a little bit. You can get fiber into your diet either through the soluble or insoluble methods.

As you can see, there are differences in the kinds of carbs that you can choose to put into your body. Some of them can cause harm to the body while others are really going to help it out. It is never safe to go on a low carb diet for a long time because it is going to end up harming you because you are missing out on important nutrients that are needed. Make sure to choose the carbs you are consuming wisely to get the best results.

Chapter 2. Why Humans Are Starch Eaters

When thinking back to how our ancestors were able to get the food that they eat, many people imagine them running around and hunting everything that they caught. It is known that the earliest of humans were not able to cultivate large fields and grow all of the foods that we enjoy today.

But when it is thought about, does it make much sense that our ancestors were running around all of the time, wasting valuable energy, to catch just a small amount of food in the grand scheme of things. What were they able to survive on in order to have the energy to catch the meat? What happened if there was no meat available at some time?

Some research has shown that the ability of our ancestors to gather and eat roots, tubers, and bulbs, is what helped them to survive and even increased the brain size of humans. Without this ability, humans would never have been able to survive and grow in order to begin living off the meat around them.

This chapter is going to focus on how humans are starch eaters and how this was able to help them to survive the sometimes harsh conditions which surrounded them while also setting them apart from other animals.

IS IT IN OUR GENES?

There is some research that believes that there is a gene that is able to produce a specific protein designed to break down any starch that is consumed into glucose that can be better used in digestion and in the body. In a paper published in *Nature Genetics* by Nathaniel Dominy, a student at ASU, this protein seems to be universal in humans. This study took samples of saliva from different populations throughout the world. It showed that those who had more copies of amylase 1 would have more of this protein that was able to turn the starch into glucose. For example, societies, such as the Japanese, that eat a lot of starches will have more copies of this particular gene compared to other groups.

This seems to suggestion that the protein could have developed through evolution. Those who still lived in areas that did not contain a lot of wild game would have to rely more of the starch digestion compared to those who were able to get other sources of food. This starch is still present in all of the populations studied, showing that starch is still a food that is common in many diets.

Why Do You Need This Gene?

You may be wondering why you would need this gene. Couldn't people have survived just fine without having this gene to help them out? Why is it so important to have this gene in order to survive?

To start with, starch is able to be converted into glucose in your body in a more natural way. It is going to slowly change and will not go into the body already in the pure form. This causes the body to work harder and will slow down the release of glucose into the brain so that it is steadier over time rather than getting it all at once. This provides your body and brain with the glucose it needs without all of the harmful effects that come with high blood sugar levels.

Another reason that it was so important for our ancestors to have this gene was because they ate a good deal of starches in their diets. It was much easier to grow a few starchy foods compared to having to prepare weapons, travel, and then hunt down an animal. Having the protein amylase 1 in their saliva allowed them to properly digest this food for their needs.

CHAPTER 3. PRO-VEGANISM

In a counter movement that is going against the popularity of the low carb, veganism has begun to grow. This is a diet plan that embraces consuming carbs, although you will need to still be careful about the types of carbs that you eat. This diet recognizes that not all carbs are bad and that you need them in order to be healthy. It also notes that you should avoid bad carbs as well as many meat sources that are harming your body just as badly if not worse than the carbs.

To learn a little more about the vegan diet and how it can be healthy for you to eat carbs in your diet, read below.

THE BASICS OF VEGANISM

A vegan diet is one that excludes any and all products that come from animals including honey, gelatin, fish, poultry, beef, eggs, and dairy. Instead, those who follow this diet, vegans, will include many foods that come from plants, whole grains, seeds, nuts, fruits, and vegetables. The staples of this diet are going to come mainly from plants and other healthy foods.

The term of vegan was first coined during the 1940s by the founder of the British Vegan Society, Donald Watson. Since that time, there has be a rise in those who follow this diet due to better understanding of human nutrition as well as the realization that eating a diet full of plant based food is great for the body.

There are many different reasons that people will choose to go on a vegan diet such as personal, environmental, and ethical health. Those who do it for ethical reasons will often extend these principles past dinner time and might also abstain from using animals for other parts of their lives such as their medicines, cosmetics, and clothing. When it comes to the ethical vegan, anything that has used animals is off limits and considered cruel.

Some are vegans because of their environment. It might be difficult to get various types of food such as meat when you live way up north or on an island that does not have enough room to grow livestock. These people will often live vegan lifestyles more out of necessity rather than choice but they are still able to get many of the same great benefits.

In America, most people will go on a vegan diet for personal reasons. They might feel that it is healthier for their bodies to do this. They might not like the taste of meat and so enjoy a diet that is full of natural and great tasting foods. Some even go on it because their favorite celebrity has endorsed the diet.

Since you will be eliminating the meats that are in your diet, you will need to get these nutrients from other sources. Often this will come from other protein sources as well as from your fruits and vegetables. While these do have carbs in them, something that is considered a bad thing in low carb diet, a vegan diet recognizes them as good and healthy and encourages you to eat them in order to stay healthy.

WHY IT IS HEALTHY

There are many health benefits that you will be able to get from a vegan diet that is balanced and healthy. Many of these benefits will not be found if you are going on a low carb diet and missing out on the nutrients that come from these foods.

To start with, a vegan diet can help you to reduce your risk of heart disease no matter which stage of your life you are in. In fact, there are many nutrition experts who recommend that those with a high risk of heart disease follow a vegan diet in order to keep it in check.

You will also be able to lose weight. When you get rid of all the extra calories that come in a vegan diet, whether that is from the meats you are consuming or from the processed foods that you are giving up, it is easier to cut down on your calorie intake and losing weight is easier.

You will also be able to lower your blood sugar levels and might find that you will be able to more effectively deal with your diabetes. This is because you are eliminating a lot of packaged foods as well as choosing more carbs that are healthier for your body rather than those that raise the blood sugar. While the vegan diet does not tell you to get rid of all the carbs you are consuming, it does ask that you consume certain ones and avoid others, which results in a healthier you.

Many people are concerned when they start on the vegan diet about whether they are going to be able to get the nutrients that their body needs. They imagine that they will just have to eat fruits and vegetables, wasting away because they are not eating what their bodies need.

If you eat a balanced vegan diet, you will still get the nutrients that your body needs. There are a lot of vegan substitutes for this diet that will ensure that you are getting the protein and other nutrients that you need. The fruits, vegetables, and other foods that you will be consuming with the vegan diet will easily help you to get the nutrients that you need, and many more than you would get from a regular diet, as long as you make sure to eat a variety of the foods during the diet.

CHAPTER 4. HIGH VS. LOW CARB ILLNESS RATES

Despite what is touted in many popular diets, eating a lot of carbs is not going to make you any unhealthier. In fact, just look at countries all over the world. Those who have what are typically considered bad eating habits, such as the French, have some of the best heart health in the whole world while others who eat more fat and fewer carbs have some of the worst. This is evident when looking at many countries like Ukraine who eat primarily animal fats.

HIGH CARBS RATES

Just because you are eating more carbs in your diet does not mean that you will be gaining weight or having to worry about other health issues. Countries such as France eat plenty of carbs and they have some of the best hearts in the world.

In research that has been done, the body is more efficiently able to digest and store fat compared to carbs. The carbs are going to be digested, used, and then disposed of if you are not able to use them all. On the other hand, the body will be able to store up any fat over and over again that you are not using, causing you to gain weight and is the leading cause of obesity in developing countries. For example, the United States consumes a ton of products that contain fat in them and they often have the highest obesity rates in the whole world. Of course, some fat is required to keep the body working efficiently, but limiting the amount and making sure to consume the right kind is necessary to prevent obesity and the other health issues that come with it.

Diabetes is another health condition you may be curious about. Many believe that by consuming too many carbs in their diet they are going to be causing more issues with diabetes if they already have it or increasing their risk of diabetes if they do not have it.

For diabetes, it is all going to depend on the type of carbs you are consuming. If you are consuming a ton of sugar each day and nothing of nutritional value, yes you will increase your risk of getting diabetes. This does not mean that all carbs are going to lead to the development of diabetes. Eating whole rains and complex carbs can actually help with preventing diabetes. The factor that is most likely to cause diabetes is the consumption of fat that is leading to obesity in many people. This extra fat storage in the body is shown to lead to higher development in diabetes compared to complex carbs and other foods.

Next is heart disease. Obesity is the main cause of many heart diseases and consuming too much fat can make the issue even worse. In countries that consume a lot of fat, like the United States, heart disease is a major concern and keeps on growing. If this diet were switched with a diet higher in carbs, healthy carbs of course, the risk of heart disease will go down and become more manageable. Reducing the amount of fat that you consume can help to keep your heart healthy for the long term.

When it comes to cancer, it is believed that eating red meat and a lot of fat are two of the most prominent risk factors of it developing in a person. On the other hand, healthy carbs such as cereal foods, vegetables, and fruits are often considered foods that can help to prevent cancer. This can be because the genetics that come with cancer will react differently with fats than they do with carbs. In addition, it has shown that obesity is linked to higher risk levels of cancer in many people.

These are just a few of the illnesses and health issues that can be caused simply by taking in too much fat in your diet. Carbs are not the enemy here; unlike what many diet plans are trying to tell you. While it is best to not eat a lot of donuts and pastries all day long and you should stick with eating the more complex forms instead, fat is often the issue that comes up when you are dealing with your health.

CHAPTER 5. RULES OF MACRONUTRIENTS

To have a good and healthy diet, it is important that you get the right amount of nutrients in the foods that you are consuming. If you eat the right kinds of foods and get the right amounts of macronutrients in each day, you will be able to stay healthy, prevent diseases, and have a great life. This chapter is going to talk about the 80/10/10 rule of macronutrients and how it can help you to get the best health results.

THE 80/10/10 RULE

The best way for you to make sure that you are getting the nutrients that your body needs is to follow the 80/10/10 rule for macronutrients. This is a simple way for you to remember the amount of each nutrient that you will need to take in for the best health.

This rule basically states that no matter how many calories that you are consuming, you should make sure that 80 percent of the calories come from carbs, 10 percent of the calories come from fat, and the other 10 percent of the calories come from protein.

The amount of each food group that you eat is going to vary depending on the amount of calories that you are consuming and so you can figure out your own recommended amounts. If you are trying to lose weight, you will just limit the amount of calories you are consuming and then calculate out your new nutrient amounts from that.

EATING THE RIGHT NUTRIENTS

It is important to realize that you still need to eat foods that are healthy for you even if you are following the right percentages of the nutrients. Just because you are allowed to have so many grams of carbs does not mean that you are able to eat anything and count it while still maintaining your health. There is balance in everything and eating the right kinds of foods within the limits is important as well.

To start with is protein. You need to consume enough protein each day to keep your muscles fed and working hard all day long. Without protein, you will find that you feel weak, are not able to do some of the tasks that you would like, and you will feel hungry more often. Protein is great for keeping the muscles going strong as well as keeping your belly full much longer.

When choosing proteins, it is recommended to choose ones that are lean such as poultry, turkey, and fish. These will have little fat but are full of the protein as well as other nutrients that your body is looking for. The best part is that with these lean sources of protein, you will not have to worry about eating a lot of extra fat and can instead choose fat from other places in your meals.

While eating a few of these meats are allowed if you are not eating a vegan diet, you should try to only eat them sparingly. Stick with sources of protein that are more plant based. These will help you to avoid the fat almost completely while still getting the carbs and the protein that your body needs.

For protein, you need to make sure to avoid red meats as much as possible. These are full of the fat that you should be avoiding and eating too much of them is going to cause heart health issues as well as obesity and other problems. Stick with the lean meats to get the best results.

Next is fat. You are allowed to consume fat in your diet, but you will need to limit it as well as making sure to consume the right kinds of fats. Bad fats, like those that you will find in fast foods, deep fried foods, and foods that are processed and easy to prepare, should be avoided at all costs.

This does not mean that all fats are bad for your body. In fact, your body needs to have some fat in it in order to work in the proper way that you would like. You should never have a diet that does not have any fat; you just need to make sure that you are limiting the amounts of fat that you are consuming as well as watching the types that you consume.

The majority of the calories that you consume should come from carbs. These are a great energy source and will keep you going strong and your body working as hard as you do. Of course, just like anything else, you will need to make sure that you are eating the right kinds of carbs. You are not going to stay very healthy if you just eat processed and simple carbs all day long because these are going to easily digest in the stomach and will spike up your blood sugar levels with a corresponding crash.

Instead, you need to make sure to choose complex carbs to make your requirements. These are full of the nutrients that your body needs to stay strong and will not cause the huge spikes in blood sugars like the simple carbs do. The complex carbs will slowly release inside the body, giving you the energy that you need without the corresponding crash. If you are able to pick out the right kinds of carbs and eat them in your meals you will be able to maintain the perfect health that you want.

In addition to these macronutrients, you should make sure that you are eating the right balance of other nutrients. A complete diet is important for overall health; regardless of how well you are doing with the macronutrients, missing out on little nutrients can harm your health as well. Take the time to plan out meals and get the right ratios of nutrients to get your best health.

Chapter 6. Negative Effects of Low Carb Diets

If you are in the market for a diet plan to help you to lose the weight that you would like, you are at some point going to come across information about a low carb diet. They seem to be everywhere and there are a lot of different versions of each. Some examples would be the Paleo diet, the south beach diet, Atkins diet, and so much more. each of these are going to have some different recommendations that you should follow for better health but all of them have one thing in common; severely limit the amounts of carbs you are consuming in order to be successful.

Despite the popularity of these diet plans, eating a low carb diet for the long term is not a healthy way for you to live. There are many negative side effects that can come with these diets. These will be discussed in more detail below.

EARLY EFFECTS

When you first start out with your low carb diet, you are forcing the body to use a different method in order to burn fat. Despite this, you will not notice a lot of side effects when you are first starting. Some of the side effects that you will notice include constipation and headache. You might also notice rashes, muscle weakness, diarrhea, and bad breath. These are often due to the fact that you are cutting out a large source of nutrients when you start out on this diet plan and your body is trying to let you know.

Mental Effects

If you continue on with the low carb diet that you have chosen, there are sometimes reports of mental effects. This is often due to the fact that your body is changing away from the use of glucose as its fuel source and instead has to rely on the use of other compounds in order to give you the energy that you need. There was one study that was done in 2009 that showed how following a low carb diet can sometimes cause memory problems that are often temporary. This is due to the fact that you are eliminating the amount of carbs out of your diet that it is used to having there. Your brain needs the carbs in order to function properly and without them, you will find that the mind is not sure how to function.

Your mood can also be influenced by the low carb diet. It has been found that while a low fat diet is able to help with the improvement of your overall mood, this is not something that is found in those who are following a diet that is low carb.

Lasting Effects

Since low carb diets are relatively new on the market, there is not a lot that is known about the long term ramifications for those who decide to stick with one of these diets for the long term. There have been a few studies done though that is used to help determine this issue.

To start with, there is a lot of research that shows how eating too much meat in your diet is able to increase your chances of developing goat, a form of arthritis that can be chronic as well as painful. Another issue that is known with low carb diets is constipation due to the fact that followers are not getting near enough of the fiber that they need. Chronic constipation could cause issues with your intestinal health and over time it could increase your risk of developing some forms of cancer.

Another problem that could happen is that a low fiber and high protein diet could over time increase the calcium amounts that are excreted through the urine. If this continues for a long time, you may start to develop kidney stones and even lead to osteoporosis.

As you can see, there are many issues that can come into effect when you are dealing with a low carb diet. While many swear that it worked for them and that it was the only way that they were able to lose the weight that they wanted, it is often considered to be really unhealthy. You are depriving your body of the nutrients that it needs in order to stay working efficiently and strong. Whenever you do this, you are causing a lot of harm to the health of your body. Eating a balanced diet is a much better way to ensure that you stay healthy compared to a diet that asks you to eliminate a lot of the healthy foods that your body needs.

CONCLUSION

Carbs are a great food source that can provide your body with a lot of the nutrients that it needs to stay healthy while also keeping the brain working efficiently. It is not a good idea to completely avoid carbs in the foods that you at, despite what many diet plans claim about how eliminating carbs will make you feel healthier. When eating the right kinds of carbs you will be able to improve your health much better than consuming a ton of fat. Use this guidebook to help better understand the importance of carbs in your overall health.